# BEGINNER GUIDE TO FIRST AID

**All You Need to Know about First Aid Treatment: Applying Bandages, Treating Cuts, Scrapes, Bleedings, Choking, Shock, Allergic Reaction, Hypothermia and Other Emergencies**

## Gloria Cornwell

# Table of Contents

# Introduction

Welcome to the basic first aid! This book will teach you the fundamentals of first aid and how to use them in a wide range of scenarios.

I have seen firsthand the positive impact that receiving first aid may have. Because I am a fireman and an emergency medical technician, I have provided first aid to a great number of individuals who were in need. I have seen firsthand how a small number of straightforward actions may contribute to the saving of lives, and it is my sincere wish that reading this book will provide you with the information and expertise necessary to do the same lifesaving work.

This book will provide you with the resources you need to be able to aid others, regardless of whether you are a medical professional or a member of the general public. It will cover the essentials of first aid, such as what to do if someone has a big wound or a small burn, in addition to the actions that need to be taken in order to deal with a suspected heart attack.

If you want to discover how to help others when they get hurt, keep reading.

# What Is First Aid?

Everyone should have some level of familiarity with first aid since it is such a crucial skill. First aid is the providing of first treatment for a sickness or injury and is often done by a person who is not trained as a medical practitioner. In the event of a crisis, having this knowledge and ability might be the difference between life and death for the person who has it.

**Fundamentals of First Aid**

The following are the primary actions involved in providing first aid:

**Assess the situation:** The first step in administering first aid is assessing the situation. Performing this step requires determining the kind and extent of the injury or sickness, as well as the number of persons affected and the setting.

**Safety:** It is essential to make certain that the protection of all those engaged is the first concern. This involves both the individual receiving the first assistance and the person delivering it.

**Call for assistance:** If required, the next step is to call for assistance. This may need contacting an ambulance, a physician, or a medical institution for assistance.

**Treatment:** Once it has been determined that the environment is safe, the affected person may then be treated. This may require administering primary emergency treatment, such as applying pressure to the wound to halt the bleeding or performing cardiopulmonary resuscitation (CPR).

**Follow-up**: After the first therapy has been administered, it is essential to check in with the person to make certain that they are continuing to get the appropriate medical care. This may require speaking with the individual's primary care physician or taking the individual to a medical institution for further treatment.

# Basic First Aid Supplies

When it comes to giving basic first aid, having the appropriate materials on hand is really necessary. Bandages, gauze, antiseptic wipes, gloves, and a thermometer are some examples of what may fall under this category. In the event of a crisis, it is essential to have a first aid bag that is not only present but also easily accessible.

In the event of an unexpected accident or medical emergency, knowing basic first aid is a skill that might make the difference between life and death. It is essential to have a working knowledge of first aid fundamentals, such as how to do an evaluation, ensure the patient's safety, summon assistance, treat the injury, and provide follow-up care. It is also vital to have the appropriate materials on hand in order to provide basic first aid to an injured person. In the event of a medical emergency, anybody who is equipped with the necessary knowledge and resources may provide first aid on a basic level.

# When Should You Use First Aid?

Knowing when and how to perform first aid in a medical emergency might be the difference between life and death. Everyone need to equip themselves with the knowledge necessary to provide first aid in case of an emergency. When someone who is wounded, unwell, or in distress needs medical aid, it is the first line of defense in delivering such assistance. This chapter will offer an overview of why first aid is essential, how to evaluate a situation, and the necessary actions to follow while delivering first aid to an injured party.

## When to Use First Aid

Assessing the situation is the first thing to do while administering first aid to someone. First, it is essential to ascertain whether or not the individual is aware and is breathing normally.

After that, an examination of any obvious injuries should be performed. If the individual is not aware or breathing, it is critical to contact 911 and begin performing cardiopulmonary resuscitation (CPR), provided that you are trained to do so. It is imperative that you phone 911 as soon as possible even if the victim is alive and breathing; but, if they have serious injuries or ones that endanger their life, it is much more critical that you do so.

First aid may be given to a person who is aware and breathing but who does not have severe or life-threatening injuries if the individual does not have any severe or life-threatening injuries. It is essential to do a thorough analysis of the circumstances and identify the most effective next steps. In these kinds of circumstances, first aid may be utilized to stop bleeding, immobilize injuries, provide comfort, and minimize swelling.

When providing first aid, it is essential to take into consideration the surrounding environment. It is important to take precautions to protect both the sufferer and the person providing first aid in the event that they are in a potentially dangerous setting, such as a crumbling building or another location with an unstable physical structure. Before administering first aid in these kinds of circumstances, it is necessary to determine the stability of the place and take measures to make it safe for people to be there.

It is also essential to take into account the degree of experience a person has when it comes to providing first aid. It is possible that a person with insufficient knowledge in first aid should not try to offer medical help in some scenarios since doing so may not be safe. In predicaments like these, it is essential to contact 911 and have a certified medical expert help you in getting back on your feet.

In the event of an emergency, having knowledge on when and how to provide first aid may save lives. It is essential to do a scenario analysis in order to ascertain the amount of medical help that is required. First aid may be given to a person who is aware and breathing, and it can be used to stop bleeding, immobilize injuries, decrease swelling, and offer comfort. It is critical to dial 911 and request help from a certified medical expert in the event that the circumstance poses a risk to one's life or the surrounding environment is dangerous. In the event of an emergency, if you know when and how to provide first aid, you may potentially assist save lives.

# Basic First Aid Procedure

This section of the book is dedicated to covering the fundamentals of first aid practice. It covers the processes that should be taken when reacting to an emergency situation, such as checking for signs of life, giving cardiopulmonary resuscitation (CPR), and using fundamental first aid treatments. In addition to this, it offers guidance on how to make appropriate use of the various first aid materials that are at your disposal, such as bandages, dressings, splints, and tourniquets. In addition, the book details how to give fundamental wound care, including how to clean and dress cuts and bruises, as well as how to identify and treat minor burns and fractures. Finally, the book offers advice on how to spot the symptoms of shock and other critical medical illnesses as well as what actions to take in response to them. Readers will finish this session with a fundamental grasp of first aid processes, as well as the information and skills required to offer basic first aid treatment. This comprehension will be accompanied by the knowledge and skills necessary to provide basic first aid care.

Bandages are an important component of first aid kits because they may be used to treat a variety of wounds and wound types. Bandages provide support, safeguard wounds, and contribute to the cessation of bleeding. In this chapter, we will explain how to use bandages in a way that is both safe and effective.

When choosing a bandage, it is important to pick one that is suitable for the kind of wound that is being treated. For instance, if you are treating a deep cut, you should use a bandage that is durable enough to cover the wound fully and is big enough to cover the area completely. When treating a minor cut, scrape, or abrasion, you should use a bandage that is thinner and less bulky.

It is important to make sure the wound is clean and dry before placing a bandage. After washing the area surrounding the wound with soap and water and blotting it dry with a clean towel, you may go on to the next step. If the wound is still bleeding, you may cover it with a gauze pad or a sterile dressing, which will both assist to staunch the bleeding and prevent further injury.

You may start applying the bandage after the wound has been well cleaned and dried. To begin, secure the bandage by wrapping it around the damaged region. The bandage should be applied in a spiral pattern around the incision, beginning at the point where the wound was opened. Make sure that the overlap between each layer of the bandage and the preceding layer is about half the width of the bandage. When you get to the end of the bandage, you should tape it so that it doesn't come undone.

When applying a bandage to a wound, you should be conscious of the pressure that the bandage might potentially provide to the wound. An excessive amount of pressure might cause more harm and impede down the healing process. If you discover that the bandage is excessively restrictive, you should take it off and rewrap it in a way that is less stringent.

After you have applied the bandage to the wound, you need to keep it on there for the duration of the healing process. The wound will be kept clean and dry, as well as protected from infection, thanks to this measure. If the bandage becomes wet or soiled, you should change it out with a new one that is clean and dry.

The use of bandages has been shown to both hasten the healing process and lower the risk of infection. The ability to properly apply bandages is an essential aspect of basic first aid, and it may be a skill that saves your life in a time of crisis if you know how to do so.

The use of dressings is an essential component of first aid. They are applied to wounds in order to cover and protect them, as well as to stop bleeding. Dressings are available in a wide range of sizes and configurations, and they may be crafted from a number of materials. Gauze, non-adherent dressings, and bandages are the three kinds of dressings that are used the most often. This is the correct way to make use of them.

**Gauze Dressings**

Gauze dressings are absorbent, so they may be used to cover wounds, keep medicine in place, and prevent infection in the wound. Before applying a gauze bandage, make sure the wound and the area around it are thoroughly cleaned with soap and water. The dressing should then be applied carefully over the wound, and either medical tape or a bandage should be used to fix it. It is possible that you may need to apply many layers of dressing to the wound if it is deep.

## Non-Adherent Dressings

Foam or fabrics are examples of the types of materials that may be used to make non-adherent dressings. They are applied to wounds in order to protect them and absorb drainage. These dressings are very helpful for wounds that are leaking or shedding fluid, so be sure you apply them in such situations. Before applying a non-adherent dressing, make sure the wound and the area around it are well cleaned with soap and water. The dressing should then be applied to the wound, and either medical tape or a bandage should be used to fix it.

## Bandages

Bandages are applied to a wound in order to provide pressure and assist control the bleeding. They also serve to maintain a dressing in place. Bandages come in a variety of shapes and sizes, the most common of which being roller bandages, triangle bandages, and elastic bandages. Before applying a bandage, make sure the wound and the area around it are thoroughly cleaned with soap and water. After that, begin wrapping the bandage around the dressing by beginning at the wound and working your way outward. Check to see that the bandage is not excessively tight, since this might restrict the flow of blood to the area. Apply medical tape or fasten the bandage in place using safety pins.

Protecting wounds and assisting in the management of bleeding are two purposes that dressings may serve. When using dressings, it is essential to first clean the wound and the area around it, then apply the dressing, and then wrap a bandage over it to keep it in place. Consult a healthcare expert for guidance on the proper application of dressings if you are unclear how to do so.

The use of a splint is an essential component of first aid at its most basic level. A splint is a piece of medical equipment that is used to immobilize and provide support for an injured limb. A bone that has been shattered may be stabilized with its help, and it can also minimize pain and edema, in addition to other issues.

Before putting a splint, it is critical to do a thorough injury assessment on the affected region as well as any additional associated wounds. Before using a splint, it is critical to stop any bleeding that may be occurring and to support the affected region if there is an open wound or a fracture. A splint may be inserted when the affected region has been stabilized.

There are a number of different splints that can be purchased, including those that are pre-made as well as those that are constructed from materials such as bandages, tape, and padding. Because they are available in a wide variety of forms and dimensions to accommodate a variety of limbs, pre-made splints are often the simplest to use. When utilizing pre-made splints, it is essential that the appropriate size and form be chosen, and that the splint be modified as required.

When treating an injury using materials such as bandages, tape, or padding, it is essential to choose the appropriate kind and size for the affected region. Before beginning to secure the splint in place with bandages, you should begin by covering the affected region with cushioning. Make sure the splint is attached securely, but avoid pulling it too tightly. Examine the patient for any indications of issues with circulation, and make any required adjustments to the splint.

After the splint has been put, it is essential to keep a close eye on the damaged region in case there are any developments. Keep an eye on the affected region for any indications of inflammation, discomfort, or other consequences. In addition to this, it is essential to examine the splint for any indications of wear and strain. If the splint has to be replaced, do it as soon as possible.

When removing a splint, it is essential to be careful and keep the damaged region supported at all times. To begin, gently pull the bands and padding apart from one another before going on to the splint itself. Make it a point to inspect the wounded region for any indications of discomfort or edema.

The use of a splint is an essential component of first aid at its most basic level. It is essential to choose the appropriate splint, both in terms of its form and size, and to carefully watch the damaged region for any signs of problems. A splint, when applied with the appropriate amount of care and attention, has the potential to make a significant contribution toward helping to alleviate pain, swelling, and other consequences.

In the event of a medical emergency, knowing how to deploy a tourniquet is an essential skill to have. Tourniquets are devices that are applied to damaged limbs in order to staunch the flow of blood. When there is serious bleeding that cannot be managed by applying direct pressure, elevating the patient, or any of the previous methods, they are utilized.

When controlling significant bleeding from a limb, tourniquets are often used. Find the damaged limb and position the tourniquet so that it is slightly above the wound. This is the first step in applying a tourniquet. Wrap the tourniquet around the affected limb and adjust it so that it is snug but not extremely so. You may fasten the tourniquet in place using a knot, a buckle, or a mechanism designed specifically for tourniquets.

Check to ensure that the tourniquet is not fastened too tightly. If it is worn excessively tightly, it might harm the tissues and prevent blood from flowing freely. It is important to make sure that the tourniquet is tight enough to stop the bleeding, but not so tight that it entirely shuts off circulation.

If the bleeding is really serious, you could be required to keep the tourniquet in place for as long as two hours. If, after two hours, the bleeding has not ceased, relax the tourniquet and then reapply it to the affected area.

Once the tourniquet has been tightened, you should seek medical treatment as soon as possible. It is essential to maintain an elevated position for the wounded leg while also monitoring the patient's vital signs.

Be cautious to go slowly and gently while removing the tourniquet from the patient's arm. It is possible that the tourniquet damaged part of the tissue, and the abrupt release of pressure may have produced an abrupt increase in the amount of bleeding.

It is essential to keep in mind that tourniquets should only be used in life-threatening emergencies. It is preferable not to use a tourniquet if the bleeding is not significant and can be controlled by applying direct pressure, elevating the affected area, and/or using other steps.

In the event of a medical emergency, tourniquets may be helpful tools; nevertheless, it is important to apply them with extreme care and only when absolutely required. In the event of a medical emergency, being able to properly apply a tourniquet may be a skill that saves lives.

# Cuts and Scrapes

Some of the most frequent types of injuries that individuals get are cuts and scrapes. [Citation needed] Everyone will experience cuts and scrapes at some point in their lives, whether they are the result of an accident in the kitchen, a tumble, or just coming into contact with a sharp item. You are in luck because there are a few easy measures you can take to assist in the prevention of infection and to ensure that the wound heals in the correct manner.

## Step 1: Clean the Wound

When treating a cut or scrape, the first thing that should be done is to clean the wound. After the injury has occurred, this step has to be taken as quickly as feasible. Begin by eliminating any potential for infection by thoroughly washing your hands. After that, give the wound a gentle rinsing with some warm water in order to eliminate any remaining dirt or debris that may be there.

## Step 2: Stop the Bleeding

After the incision has been cleansed, it is imperative that the bleeding be stopped. Applying direct pressure to the wound with a clean cloth or bandage for a few minutes is the first step in treating it. Seek medical care immediately in the event that the bleeding does not stop.

## Step 3: Apply Antibiotic Ointment

After ensuring that there is no more loss of blood, it is time to apply an antibiotic ointment. This will prevent the wound from being inflamed and will also help prevent it from becoming infected. Make sure that just a little amount of the ointment is applied to the wound, but that it is well covered.

## Step 4: Dress the Wound

Following the application of the ointment, a bandage or a sterile gauze pad should be placed over the wound. This will assist in keeping the wound clean and preventing the entry of germs. Make sure the bandage is changed at least once a day, or anytime it gets filthy or wet, whichever occurs first.

## Step 5: Keep an Eye on the Wound

It is essential to maintain a close check on the wound to ensure that it is healing in the correct manner. In the event that the incision becomes red, swells up, or begins to leak pus, it is possible that it is infected and you should seek medical assistance as soon as possible.

The majority of injuries, such as cuts and scratches, are easily treated at home with only a few basic steps. You can assist ensure that the wound heals correctly and fast by thoroughly cleansing the wound, halting any bleeding that may be occurring, administering antibiotic ointment to the wound, covering the wound, and keeping an eye out for any symptoms of infection.

# Burns

Burns are an extremely frequent kind of injury that may lead to potentially severe complications. It is essential to have knowledge of the procedures to follow in the event that someone is suffering from a burn. In this chapter, we will cover the fundamentals of administering first aid for burns, including how to determine the extent of the burn and how to effectively treat it. In addition to that, it will provide a general review of when and how one should seek medical treatment.

## Assessing the Severity of Burns

The first thing that has to be done in order to provide first aid for burns is to determine how severe the burn is. Redness, swelling, and discomfort are the three most common symptoms associated with minor burns. Burns of the first degree are the most dangerous kind and may cause the skin to blister. Burns of the second degree are more severe than burns of the first degree and cause the skin to seem moist, glossy, and blistering. Burns of the third degree are the most severe. They leave the skin scorched or white, and the victim is no longer responsive to touch.

## Burns: Treating Minor Burns

If the burn is just mild, the first step is to cool it by running cold or lukewarm water over it for 10 to 15 minutes. If the burn is severe, the next step is to seek medical attention. Do not apply ice to the skin since it might result in more harm. After the burn has had a chance to cool, a sterile bandage or cloth need to be applied on top of it. To alleviate the discomfort, it is possible to use painkillers that are available without a prescription.

## Burns: Treating Serious Burns

If the burn is more serious, it is essential to get medical assistance as soon as you can after experiencing it. There is a risk of infection if you use ointments, lotions, butter, or any other home remedy. Avoid applying them. Take off any clothes or jewelry that is either directly on top of or near the burn, but be cautious not to pull off any items that are firmly adhered to the wound. Cover the burn with a sterile bandage or fabric that does not adhere to the wound. Never apply direct pressure to the burn or burst any blisters that may have formed.

## When Should You Seek Medical Attention for Burns

It is important to get medical assistance as soon as possible if the burn is severe, covers more than 10 percent of the body, is deep, or is located on the face, hands, feet, or groin region. In addition, prompt medical treatment should be sought out in the event that the individual starts to develop symptoms such as disorientation, nausea, or dizziness.

Burns may vary from being quite harmless to life-threatening, therefore it is essential to be aware of how to determine the extent of a burn and how to treat it appropriately. When dealing with mild burns, it is vital to wrap the affected area with a clean bandage or cloth, apply cold or lukewarm water to the burn for ten to fifteen minutes, and take over-the-counter pain medicine if required. When dealing with burns of a more severe kind, quick medical assistance is required. A person may assist ensure that they get the appropriate care and treatment and prevent any significant consequences by being familiar with the actions that need to be taken for burn treatment.

# Broken bones

Fractures, which are another name for broken bones, are one of the most frequent types of injuries and may vary from being very mild to being quite serious. It is crucial to be knowledgeable about how to treat a fracture in order to reduce the likelihood of further injuries or problems. This chapter will give a step-by-step instruction on how to correctly address a fracture, beginning with the first examination and continuing all the way through getting medical assistance.

## Step 1: Determine the extent of the injury

The first thing that has to be done is an examination of the injury. Keep an eye out for telltale indicators of shattered bones, such as an evident deformity or the inability to move the limb that's been injured. Check for any further injuries that may be related with it, such as cuts, bruises, or swelling. If the individual is aware, you should inquire about the level of pain and any other symptoms they may be experiencing.

## Step 2: Stop the Bleeding

Applying direct pressure with a clean cloth or bandage to the incision is important to stop any bleeding that may be occurring. Raise the leg so that it is higher above the level of the heart in order to slow or stop the flow of blood. Do not use a tourniquet since doing so might result in even more severe injuries.

## Step 3: Make sure the Limb Cannot Move

In order to prevent any more injury, the limb will now need to be immobilized. Make use of a splint or another firm object such as a towel or newspaper that has been rolled up to assist in holding the limb in place. Be certain that the splint does not apply any pressure to the broken bone and that the limb retains some range of motion even while it is immobilized.

**Step 4: Seek Professional Medical Help**

After you have successfully immobilized the limb, you should seek medical assistance as quickly as you can. It is essential to keep in mind that a bone that has been shattered in any form should not be moved or manipulated in any way, as doing so might result in more damage to the bone.

Fractures, also known as broken bones, may vary from being quite small to being quite serious. In order to reduce the likelihood of subsequent damage or problems, it is important to handle fractures correctly. This chapter offered a step-by-step tutorial on how to appropriately deal with a fracture, beginning with the first examination and continuing all the way through to obtaining medical assistance. You may assist guarantee the person who fractured their bone gets the

highest level of treatment possible by adhering
to the steps that are provided in this guide and
using them.

# Bleedings

The occurrence of bleeding is a frequent and significant medical problem that requires prompt attention and cautious consideration. It might be the consequence of a little injury like a cut or scrape, or it could be the result of a more catastrophic accident like a fractured bone or a deep wound. In any event, it is essential to take the required precautions to stop the bleeding and get medical help if necessary. This article will offer an introduction to the procedures that should be followed when someone is bleeding.

## Putting a Stop to the Bleeding

When dealing with an injury that is causing bleeding, the first thing that has to be done is to stop the bleeding. When treating a cut of this severity, a simple pressure bandage should do the trick. Put direct pressure on the wound using a clean cloth or bandage for a few minutes, or until the bleeding stops completely, whichever comes first. If the cut is more significant or if applying pressure does not stop the bleeding, a tourniquet may be required to halt the bleeding. Because improper application or prolonged use of a tourniquet may result in severe tissue damage or even the amputation of a limb, it should only be used in the most extreme emergencies.

## Taking Care of the Wound

The following step, which should be taken when the bleeding has been stopped, is to clean the wound. To wipe away any grime or particles, all you need is a fresh towel and some hot water. If the wound is significant, it is possible that it may need irrigating with a sterile solution. If the wound is filthy or infected, it has to be treated using a disinfectant such hydrogen peroxide or iodine so that it can heal properly.

## Putting Bandages on the Cut

After the wound has been cleansed, a dressing should be put to it so that it is protected from becoming infected. Pick a dressing that is big enough to cover not just the wound but also the region immediately around it. Bandages or medical tape may be used to keep the dressing in place. It is important to get medical assistance as soon as possible if the wound is severe or needs stitches.

**Keeping an Eye on the Injury**

After the wound has been cleaned and bandaged, it is critical to observe it closely for any indications that it may have become infected. Examine the wound on a regular basis for any indications of infection, such as redness, swelling, discharge, or any other symptoms. Seek medical assistance as soon as possible if any of these symptoms appear.

Bleeding is a frequent and significant medical condition that requires quick attention from a healthcare provider. If you take the required precautions to stop the bleeding, clean the wound, and patch it, you may help reduce the likelihood of developing an infection or experiencing any other consequences. In the event that the bleeding is serious or does not stop when pressure is applied, you should seek medical treatment as soon as you can. By adhering to these fundamental principles, it is feasible to treat a bleeding injury in a timely manner while minimizing the risk of further complications.

# Choking

A medical emergency that demands urgent care and must be regarded extremely seriously is choking. This condition should not be taken lightly. If prompt medical attention is not received and provided in the appropriate manner, choking may sometimes result in significant injuries or even fatalities. Learning what to do in order to save someone's life in the case that they are choking on anything is very important. Helping someone who is choking may be done in a series of steps, which will be outlined in this article.

## Step 1: Determine if the individual is choking

When someone looks to be choking, the first thing that should be done is to verify that they are, in fact, choking. Even if someone is coughing or producing other sounds, it does not mean that they are unable to breathe. If, on the other hand, a person is unable to produce any sound at all, it is quite probable that they are choking and need more aid.

## Step 2: Ask if the Person is Choking

If the individual is unable to produce any sounds, you should inquire as to whether or not they are choking. If they are able to reply, it is quite probable that they are not choking and that they may be able to throw up the item on their own. If they are unable to react, however, it is likely because they are choking and need assistance.

## Step 3: Perform the Heimlich Maneuver

If it seems that the individual is having difficulty breathing, the next thing to do is the Heimlich technique. Standing behind the victim, placing your arms around their waist, and forming a fist with one hand are the steps involved in this technique. Position your fist so that it is just over the individual's belly button, then use your other hand to grip it. Make sure that your arms are straight the whole time, and then use fast, strong actions to drive upward and inward. Continue doing this until the foreign item has been ejected.

## Step 4: Call 911

In the event that the individual is still unable to breathe, contact 911 as soon as possible. Maintaining the Heimlich technique is necessary until assistance is received.

The medical condition known as choking is considered a significant emergency and needs quick care. Understanding what to do in an emergency situation when someone is choking might be the difference between life and death. You may be able to help save the life of someone who is choking on something by following the instructions that have been detailed for you above. If the item is not ejected after many attempts, you should not hesitate to phone 911.

# Heat related emergencies

Emergencies brought on by heat are a significant reason for worry since they may lead to severe disease, injury, or even death in extreme circumstances. Emergencies connected to heat may happen if someone is exposed to high temperatures for a long period of time, does not drink enough water, and does not take the appropriate cooling measures. It is necessary to have knowledge of the signs and symptoms of heat-related crises, as well as how to react to them, in order to protect the health and safety of individuals who are impacted.

**Step 1: Recognize the signs and symptoms**

Recognizing the signs and symptoms of a heat-related emergency is the first step in developing a response to the situation. The majority of people who have this condition will experience excessive sweating, dizziness, nausea, disorientation, muscular cramps, fast breathing and pulse rate, and even fainting. In the event that any of these symptoms are present, it is imperative that action be taken as soon as possible.

## Step 2: Get the affected person out of the heat

The second thing that has to be done is to get the individual who is being affected out of the heat as quickly as possible. This may be accomplished by relocating them to a location that is shady, cool, and perhaps even air-conditioned, if one is available. If the individual is unable to move, you may give some respite from the heat by using a fan or damp cloths to cool them down.

## Step 3: Loosen or remove any clothes that needs to be adjusted

The third stage is to adjust the individual's clothes such that there is less of a restriction on the passage of air and less of an increase in the person's core temperature. This may assist in lowering the temperature of the body and bringing about some degree of comfort.

## Step 4: Provide hydration

The injured individual should be given some fluids as the fourth stage in the process. You may do this by providing them with refreshing water or a sports drink to help replace their lost electrolytes. If the individual is unable to drink, you may saturate their skin with cold water or apply damp towels on the back of their neck and under their armpits to help them stay hydrated.

## Step 5: Seek the Attention of a Medical Professional

If the individual does not exhibit any indications of improvement, the fifth and last step is to seek professional medical assistance. Emergencies brought on by heat may be quite dangerous; in extreme situations, they can even lead to death. Serious disease, injury, or both can result.

Emergencies brought on by heat may be quite dangerous; in extreme situations, they can even lead to death. Serious disease, injury, or both can result. It is necessary to have knowledge of the signs and symptoms of heat-related crises, as well as how to react to them, in order to protect the health and safety of individuals who are impacted. In the case of a heat-related emergency, being sure to follow the actions that are indicated in this guidance may assist to guarantee that a prompt and efficient response is provided.

# Allergic Reaction

An allergic reaction takes place when the body's natural defenses have an exaggerated response to a material that would normally be considered safe, such as pollen, peanuts, or shellfish. Allergic responses may vary from being very harmless to being extremely dangerous, and in rare instances, they can even be fatal. It is essential to have a fundamental understanding of how to manage allergic reactions, as well as the signs and symptoms of an allergic response, in order to provide basic first aid.

**Step-by-Step Guide**

1. Perform a thorough examination looking for indications and symptoms of an allergic response. Symptoms such as hives, itching, swelling, asthma, trouble breathing, coughing, vomiting, stomach discomfort, and loss of consciousness are all possible reactions.

2. If the individual is aware, you should inquire as to whether or not they are allergic to anything and whether or not they are in possession of any medicine, such as an EpiPen or an antihistamine.

3. If the individual has access to medicine, assist them in taking it in accordance with the directions printed on the label.

4. Make an instant call to either 911 or the emergency medical services in your area if the individual is experiencing severe symptoms and does not have access to any medicine to treat them.

5. While the individual is waiting for medical assistance, ensure that they are as comfortable as possible. Relax any constricting garments and put the person in a posture that will make it simpler for them to breathe, such as sitting in an upright position.

6. If the individual is experiencing trouble breathing, a rescue inhaler should be administered if one is available.

7. If the individual is throwing up, make sure they are in a posture that will protect them from choking on their own vomit.

8. Do not offer the individual anything to eat or drink since doing so may cause the symptoms to become much more severe.

9. Keep an eye on the person's respiration as well as their pulse.

Allergic responses may vary from being very harmless to being extremely dangerous, and in rare instances, they can even be fatal. It is essential to have a fundamental understanding of how to manage allergic reactions, as well as the signs and symptoms of an allergic response, in order to provide basic first aid. You may assist in keeping someone safe until medical assistance comes if you follow the instructions that have been explained above.

# Treating shock

Shock is a condition that poses a significant risk to a person's life and needs quick medical intervention. This condition is brought on by a dramatic drop in blood pressure, which in turn causes a reduction in the supply of oxygen to the cells and organs of the body. Shock is a potentially life-threatening medical condition that may be brought on by a variety of conditions and injuries, including extreme bleeding, allergic responses, burns, dehydration, and severe physical trauma. To effectively treat shock, one must first have a knowledge of the underlying cause of the condition and then take immediate measures to stabilize the patient before obtaining professional medical assistance.

## Evaluation and Stabilization

The first treatment for shock consists of evaluating the patient's status and taking any necessary actions to stabilize them. To begin, check all of your vital signs, including your pulse, your respiration, and your blood pressure. If the patient is aware, you should interrogate them to discover whether or not they are in a state of shock. For instance, you may inquire as to whether or not they are experiencing chest discomfort, shortness of breath, or dizziness. Perform a thorough examination of the patient, looking for indications of shock such as pale complexion, reduced urine production, and fast breathing.

Take the necessary precautions to stabilize the patient if there are any indications that they may be going into shock. Place the patient in a relaxed seated posture and raise their feet about 12 inches off of the ground. Because of this, blood flow to both the heart and the brain will be improved. If the patient is shivering, wrapping them with a blanket will allow them to retain more of their body heat.

**Taking Care of the Root of the Problem**

Finding out what caused the shock in the first place and addressing that condition is the next stage in the treatment process. If the patient is experiencing hypovolemic shock as a result of significant bleeding, direct pressure should be applied to the wound using a sterile dressing. In the event that an allergic response is detected, epinephrine should be given as soon as it is practicable. If the patient has an open wound, an antibiotic ointment should be used, and then the wound should be dressed. In order to effectively treat shock, it is necessary to address the underlying cause of the condition.

**Fluid Replacement**

Replacement of lost fluids is often a critical component of treating shock. This may be accomplished by administering intravenous fluids to the patient, such as lactated ringers or regular saline solution. Increasing the amount of blood that is present in the body and enhancing the flow of blood are both goals of the treatment known as fluid replacement. In situations when significant bleeding has caused hypovolemic shock, the replenishment of lost fluids is of utmost importance.

## Medication

It's possible that you'll need medication in order to treat shock. It is possible to raise blood pressure and boost blood flow with the help of several medications, including inotropes and vasopressors. It is possible to treat allergic responses with a variety of drugs, including antihistamines, for example.

Shock is a condition that puts a person's life in danger and needs immediate medical attention. The first stage in treating shock is to evaluate the patient's state and then take any necessary measures to stabilize them. It is important to determine what triggered the shock in the first place and address it. The treatment for shock may also include the administration of drugs and the restoration of fluids. When treating someone who is in a state of shock, it is essential to get medical assistance as quickly as possible.

# Hypothermia

In the medical condition known as hypothermia, the core temperature of the body dips below the usual range of 36.5 degrees Celsius (97.7 degrees Fahrenheit). As a result of the severity of the disease, prompt medical intervention is essential. If the hypothermic patient is not treated, the condition might progress to coma and ultimately result in death. Everyone is at risk for hypothermia, but the elderly, small children, and adults who stay out in the cold for extended periods of time are more likely to get the condition than others. It is essential to have the knowledge necessary to identify the signs of hypothermia as well as the appropriate treatment for it.

## Procedures to Follow When Treating Hypothermia

**1. Perform a check of the individual's vital signs:** Check the individual's temperature as well as their heart rate and respiration rate. Hypothermia is diagnosed when a person's core temperature falls below 35 degrees Celsius (95 degrees Fahrenheit).

**2. Take off wet clothes**: Take off any damp clothing that the individual is wearing and replace it with warm clothing that is dry. Cover the individual with blankets and make sure their head is hidden as well if they are unconscious.

**3. Transfer the individual to a warm and dry environment as soon as feasible**: Transfer the individual to a warm and dry environment as soon as possible. As the individual may get overheated if the atmosphere is too hot, it is important to make sure that it is not too hot.

**4. Warm the individual gradually:** Wrap the person in warm blankets or use a heating pad to gently warm them up. Burns may occur if direct heat or hot water is applied to the individual, therefore avoid doing any of those things.

**5. Provide the individual with warm fluids:** Provide the individual with warm fluids that do not include alcohol, such as tea, soup, or juice. This will assist in warming them up on the inside as well as the outside.

**6. Keep checking the individual's vital signs:** Check the individual's temperature, as well as their heart and respiration rates on a frequent basis. Check to see that the individual's temperature is rising in a measured manner and that their vital signs are not changing.

**7. Seek medical treatment:** If the individual does not improve or their vital signs worsen, seek medical assistance right away.

Hypothermia is a life-threatening medical illness that has to be attended to and treated as soon as possible. It is essential to be able to identify the signs of hypothermia and to immediately begin treatment for the condition. Seek prompt medical assistance if the condition of the individual does not improve or if there is a deterioration in the patient's vital signs. The individual who has hypothermia may make a complete recovery if they get care as soon as possible.

# Emergency Child Birth

Emergency delivery is an unforeseen and unexpected occurrence. Many women are unprepared for it, and it may be a very stressful and terrifying experience. Knowing how to handle an emergency delivery might help you be prepared if the circumstance comes.

## Step 1: Call 911

The first action to do when someone is having an emergency delivery is to contact 911. This is vital because it will assure that medical aid is on the way. If you are alone, contact 911 first, then follow the procedures below.

## Step 2: Get Supplies

The next stage is to ready supplies. You will need a clean, flat surface, like a bed or blanket, some clean towels or cloths, a thread or shoelace, and some warm water.

## Step 3: Prepare the Setting

Once you have acquired the items, prepare the atmosphere for delivery. Make sure the space is clean and free of any debris. Make an effort, if at all feasible, to ensure that the space is as pleasant and cozy as you possibly can.

## Step 4: Position the Individual

After the setting has been prepared, the individual should be put in the position to deliver. Have them lay down on their backs with their knees bent and their legs spread apart if at all feasible. In the event that this cannot be accomplished, you should have them sit up straight while leaning forward into something for support.

## Step 5: Support the individual

As soon as the individual is in the appropriate posture, you may start providing both mental and physical assistance. Talk in a level-headed and soothing manner. Instruct them to take deep breaths and concentrate on the motion of pushing.

## Step 6: Catch the Baby

When it becomes clear where the infant is, get some clean cloths or towels to use as a net to capture the child. It's possible that the baby's head and body will need to be supported when they are being delivered.

## Step 7: Tie Off the Umbilical Cord

After the baby has been delivered, the umbilical chord should be tied off with the thread or shoelace. At a distance of approximately two inches from the baby's belly, tie it safely but not too firmly.

## Step 8: Cut the Umbilical Cord

After the string has been knotted, a pair of clean scissors should be used to cut the cord in between the two knots. In order to avoid getting an infection, make sure the scissors are clean.

**Step 9: Wash the Baby**

After the umbilical chord has been cut, carefully clean the newborn with the warm water and the fresh towels. Be careful to clean the baby's body thoroughly by removing any mucous and other fluids that may be present.

The experience of giving birth in an unexpected circumstance may be stressful and terrifying. On the other hand, being aware of how to handle an unexpected delivery might help you be more prepared in the event that it occurs. If you follow the procedures that have been explained for you above, you will be in a position to be ready to offer the essential care and assistance to guarantee a safe birth.

# Spinal injuries

Spinal injuries may be very debilitating and even fatal in certain cases. They have the potential to result in death as well as lasting paralysis or impairment. As a result of this, it is essential to have a fundamental understanding of how to care for a person who has had a spinal injury. In the case of a spinal injury, this article will provide an overview of the fundamentals of first aid, including the measures to take and procedures to adhere to in the event of an emergency.

## Examining the Situation

The first action in dealing with a spinal injury is to evaluate the site of the accident. Check to see that the place is secure and that there is nothing in the vicinity that might cause the individual any additional harm. If the individual is within a car, you should not attempt to relocate them until the vehicle has been stabilized and all potential dangers have been eliminated.

## Perform a Damage Assessment

After the perimeter has been secured, the next step is to evaluate the severity of the injury. Check for any indications of trouble breathing, as well as evidence of paralysis and loss of sensation in the limbs, especially the arms and legs. If the individual is cognizant, you should urge them to move their arms and legs, and you should take note of any movement or lack of movement that they make.

## Stabilize the Neck

Following the evaluation of the damage, the following step is to stabilize the neck and spine. To do this, the patient is carefully turned over onto their back, and the neutral alignment of their neck and spine is checked before continuing. This indicates that the head should be held vertically, and there should be no bending at the angle of the neck. To do this, position your hands on each side of the person's head and apply a little amount of pressure to the top of their head while pressing it into the ground. Alternately, you might use a rolled-up towel or blanket to support the head; in this case, however, you would want to make sure that it does not put any pressure on the neck.

## Immobilize the Spine

The following phase, which occurs after the head and neck have been stabilized, is to immobilize the spine. As a means of preventing the individual from making any additional movements, this is accomplished by draping a blanket or some other cloth across the back and neck of the individual. It is essential to keep in mind that the individual should not be relocated unless it is really required to do so.

## Request Help

Call for assistance as soon as the patient's condition has been brought under control and they have their spine immobilized. Make a call to 911 or to the emergency services in your area and describe the situation to them. Provide them with precise instructions to the area and let them know that the individual may have suffered a spinal injury.

**Prepare Yourself**

Be ready for the paramedics to take control of the situation once the emergency services arrive at the scene. In the interim, make sure the individual is as comfortable as you can and refrain from moving them unless it is absolutely essential to do so.

Spinal injuries may be life-threatening and catastrophic, but it is feasible to give help in the case of an emergency if the appropriate information and first aid skills are possessed. You will be able to assist in stabilizing the neck and spine if you follow the measures given above, and you will also be able to telephone for assistance. First and foremost, keep in mind

that you should never move the individual
unless it is absolutely required.

# Poisoning

Accidental ingestion, inhalation, or skin contact with a deadly chemical may lead to poisoning, which is a frequent medical emergency that can occur in a variety of ways. If you have reason to believe that someone is poisoned, it is imperative that you be aware of how to proceed in this potentially catastrophic situation. In this chapter, we will go over the signs and symptoms of poisoning, as well as the processes for how to react to someone who has been poisoned.

## Signs and Symptoms of Poisoning

The indications of poisoning vary according to the kind of the toxin that has been swallowed, breathed in, or come into contact with the body, as well as the quantity of the toxin that has done so. The following is a list of some of the general signs and symptoms of poisoning:

- Confusion

- Nausea as well as throwing up

- Diarrhea

- Dizziness

- Abdominal discomfort

- Difficulty breathing

- Loss of consciousness

- Seizures

- Skin irritation or burns

- Loss of consciousness

## Recognizing Poisoning

It is imperative that prompt action be taken if there is even the remotest possibility that someone has been poisoned. Recognizing the signs and symptoms of poisoning is the first step in antidoting its effects. In addition, it is essential to identify the origin of the toxin, since this will assist in directing the appropriate reaction.

It is crucial to seek for any containers, spilled chemicals, or other indicators that can offer clues as to what might have caused the poisoning, especially if the origin of the poison is unclear. If you are able to identify the origin of the poison, it is imperative that you make a note of the name of the chemical as well as its concentration, as this information will be helpful in choosing the therapy that should be administered.

## What to Do in the Event of Poisoning

It is imperative that you act swiftly and seek medical assistance if you have any reason to believe that someone has been poisoned. There are a few steps you may do to aid the individual who has been poisoned while you wait for medical assistance to arrive at the scene.

1. Make certain that the individual is located in a secure area.

2. Check to see whether the individual is choking on their own vomit if they have just thrown up.

3. Keep an eye on the person's pulse and respiration rate.

4. If the individual is aware, you should start giving them water to assist prevent them from becoming dehydrated.

5. If the individual is unconscious, the recovery posture should be used on them.

6. If you are aware of the substance that caused the victim's poisoning, look for the container it came in and bring it with you when you go to the hospital.

7. If you have any idea what kind of poison it is or how much of it was ingested, you should share that information with the medical staff who are treating you.

Poisoning is a potentially dangerous medical issue that may even endanger a person's life. It is critical to have a plan in place and be aware of what to do in the event that you believe that someone has been poisoned. Helping someone who has been poisoned requires many stages, the most significant of which are recognizing the signs and symptoms of poisoning, locating the source of the poison, and taking the proper action to treat the poisoning. It is imperative that you seek medical attention as soon as possible if you have any reason to believe that someone has been poisoned.

# Bites and Stings from Animals

Being attacked by an animal may be a terrible experience, particularly if you are unprepared for how to respond in the event that you are bitten or stung. Having the knowledge to take the appropriate actions in the time may assist to lessen the likelihood of an infection occurring, as well as providing instant relief from the agony and suffering that accompany an occurrence of this kind. This chapter will give a detailed guide for dealing with animal bites and stings, and it will address the appropriate procedures that need to be taken in order to limit the danger of infection.

## First Steps

In the event that an animal has bitten or stung a person, the first thing that should be done is to evaluate the situation. It is essential that the human leave the location if the animal is still there since they might be in danger. When dealing with a potentially dangerous creature like a snake, it is critical to make every effort to determine the species if at all feasible. It is essential to determine the extent of the harm even if the animal in question is no longer present. In the event that the bite or sting is serious, it is imperative that you phone 911 as soon as possible.

**Taking Care of the Wound**

After the injured party has been evacuated from the location in a secure manner and an evaluation of the extent of their injuries has been completed, the following step is to clean the wound. When cleaning the wound, it is essential to make use of soap and water that is warm. When cleansing the wound, it is essential to be gently, since vigorous washing may result in more harm to the patient. After the wound has been thoroughly cleansed, it is necessary to re-rinse it with clean water and then pat it dry with a clean towel.

## Care for the Cut or Scrape

After the wound has been cleansed, it is necessary to treat the wound in order to lessen the likelihood of an infection occurring. It is possible that you may need to seek medical assistance, but this will depend on the severity of the cut. It is essential to apply a topical antibiotic ointment to the area, and then cover it with a clean bandage. This should be done even if the wound is not very serious. It is essential to replace the bandage every day and closely inspect the site for any indications of infection.

## Discomfort and Swelling

When an animal bites or stings a person, it is not uncommon for the victim to suffer pain and swelling in the affected area. It is essential to apply an ice pack to the affected region for a period of 15 to 20 minutes at a time in order to alleviate the discomfort and swelling. To avoid getting frostbite, it is essential to not place the ice pack directly on the skin but rather to use a towel as a barrier between the ice pack and the skin.

## Vaccinations

It is essential to seek medical assistance as soon as possible in the case that you have been bitten by an animal that has the potential to transmit rabies. In such a scenario, it is quite possible that the individual will be required to get rabies vaccination. It is critical to be vaccinated against rabies as quickly as possible after being bitten by an animal, since rabies vaccinations are readily accessible at almost all medical institutions.

The experience of being bitten or stung by an animal may be terrifying; but, if you are prepared and take the appropriate measures, you can lessen the likelihood of developing an infection and get some relief from the agony and suffering. It is essential to do an evaluation of the circumstance and remove the human from the location if the animal is still there. In addition to this, it is essential to clean the wound, treat it, and put an ice pack to it in order to alleviate the pain and swelling. Last but not least, if you have been bitten by an animal that might have rabies, you should seek medical assistance right once and be vaccinated against the disease. Rabies can be fatal.

# Disaster Reaction

The process of catastrophe management as a whole includes the disaster response process as one of its most important components. In the aftermath of a natural catastrophe or another kind of cataclysmic event, it refers to the series of steps that are done to safeguard the lives and property of individuals who have been impacted and to swiftly restore the services that are required. The reaction to a disaster may take many different shapes and include both the public and commercial sectors. The process starts with an initial evaluation of the situation, followed by the deployment of individuals and resources to meet any urgent requirements that have arisen.

**Step-by-Step Procedure**

**1. Determine the nature of the catastrophe and the breadth of its**

**effects**: The first stage in reacting to a natural or man-made disaster is to determine the nature of the event, its scale, and the geographic region that it impacts. This will assist decide the extent to which the answer that is expected must be given.

**2. Activate resources**: After it has been determined how extensive the crisis is, the following stage is to activate the individuals and resources that are required in order to provide a response. This can include local emergency responders, troops from the National Guard, or perhaps additional resources provided by the government.

**3. Establish a command structure:** One of the most important aspects of an efficient reaction is the development of a command organization. It should include representatives from all of the numerous organizations and agencies that are reacting to the situation, as well as any communities who have been impacted.

**4. Fulfill Basic needs**: The emphasis of the reaction should be on meeting the people impacted by the disaster's basic requirements, such as providing them with food, water, shelter, medical attention, and emotional support.

**5. Securing the area:** In the majority of situations, it will be required to secure the area that is impacted in order to protect individuals who are affected and to safeguard the safety of those who are responding.

**6. Analyze and prioritize needs:** Once the fundamental requirements of those impacted have been satisfied, the response must assess and prioritize the needs of the affected population.

7. **Offer support services:** In many situations, extra support services, including as search and rescue, the disposal of debris, and the reestablishment of key services, will be required.

8. **Plan for the long term**: Once the urgent requirements have been met, it is critical to begin preparing for the long-term rehabilitation of the afflicted region. This involves determining the extent of the damage, coming up with a recovery strategy, and locating the resources necessary to carry out the strategy.

The process of managing disasters as a whole includes an extremely important step called disaster response. It refers to the series of steps that are conducted in the aftermath of a catastrophic occurrence in order to safeguard the lives and property of individuals who have been impacted and to swiftly restore services that are necessary for survival. The mobilization of personnel and resources, the establishment of a command structure, the provision of basic needs, the securing of the affected area, the assessment and prioritization of needs, the provision of support services, and the planning for long-term recovery are all necessary components of an effective response. Responders may assist protect the safety and well-being of persons impacted by the catastrophe, as well as limit the long-term effects of the disaster, by following these procedures throughout the response effort.

# Preparing for Emergency

Emergencies might happen when we least anticipate them to appear in our lives. Natural catastrophes, accidents, and other unanticipated occurrences may all be the root cause of these problems. It is critical to have a plan in place for dealing with any kind of unexpected event, as this will allow you to act promptly and effectively. The crucial information that you need to prepare for an emergency, such as the measures you should take, the supplies that you should have on hand, and the procedures that you should do during an emergency, will be provided to you in this book.

## Actions to Take in Order to Be Ready for Any Emergencies

## Step 1: Create an emergency plan

Creating a strategy is the first stage in becoming ready for a crisis or unexpected event. This plan need to contain certain actions on the user's part that ought to be taken in the case of an emergency. Make sure to include your family's and friends' contact information, as well as the information for the local emergency services. You also need to include a strategy for evacuating the building and an emergency supply bag.

## Step 2: Gather Materials

In the event of a crisis, you should always have a kit for emergencies ready and waiting. This kit need to include vital items like as water, food, first aid materials, a flashlight, a whistle, and any prescriptions that you may want in the event of an emergency.

## Stage 3: Run Through Your Strategy

After you have formulated your strategy and amassed your resources, the next step is to put your strategy into action via rehearsal. You will get more acquainted with the procedures and materials you will need in the event of an emergency if you do this. You should also go through any evacuation drills that you may have prepared.

## Step 4: Keep up-to-date

It is essential that you maintain a level of awareness on any possible disasters that may be happening in your region. Either keeping up with the local news or subscribing to an emergency alert service is a good way to accomplish this goal.

## Step 5: Put Your Plan Into Motion

It is imperative that prompt action be taken in the event that an emergency does arise. Be careful to carry out the steps outlined in your plan and make use of the items included in your emergency kit. In the event that you are required to evacuate, be sure to do it in a methodical and organized way.

It is critical to ensure that you are well-prepared in case of an emergency. You will be able to react swiftly and effectively to any emergency scenario with its assistance. You will be able to handle any crisis that may arise if you follow the instructions described in this book. Create a strategy for dealing with emergencies, stock up on supplies, go through drills to become familiar with the plan, keep informed, and be prepared to respond if one does arise. You can be ready for any situation as long as you have the appropriate preparedness.

# First Aid Supplies

When it comes to giving basic first aid, having the appropriate materials on hand is really necessary. Items that are included in a person's first aid kit are those that may be used to treat minor injuries and illnesses in a prompt and efficient manner. Bandages, gauze, antiseptics, and other items for treating wounds, scratches, bruises, and sprains may be included with them. It is crucial to get acquainted with all of the required materials and know how to utilize them in order to be prepared for any first aid crisis that may arise.

**First Aid Supplies**

## 1. Bandages

Bandages are an essential component of first aid kits since they are used to both cover and safeguard wounds. There is a wide variety of bandages available, and some of the options include adhesive bandages, gauze wraps, and elastic bandages. Stick-on bandages are a convenient, time-saving option for covering up small wounds such as cuts, scrapes, and scratches. It is common practice to use adhesive bandages in combination with gauze wraps for treating bigger wounds. Gauze wraps are used to cover larger wounds. Injured parts, such as a sprained ankle or wrist, are often wrapped with elastic bandages, which offer support and stability to the affected region.

## 2. Antiseptics

Antiseptics are used to assist in the cleaning of wounds and to keep them from becoming infected. Iodine, rubbing alcohol, and hydrogen peroxide are just examples of the many kinds of antiseptics that may be found in the marketplace. Antiseptics of every kind are put to use to assist in the cleaning of and protection against infection in small wounds and scrapes.

3. Gauze: Gauze is a sort of cloth that is often applied to wounds in order to cover and protect them. It is normally constructed out of cotton or a synthetic material, and it may be purchased in a wide variety of sizes and forms. As an additional layer of protection and support for wounds, gauze is often used in conjunction with adhesive bandages and elastic bandages in many medical settings.

4. Tape: Bandages and gauze may be more securely adhered to the skin with the help of tape. Tapes are available in a variety of different forms, including those made of fabric, paper, and plastic. Cloth tape is often used in the process of adhering gauze and elastic bandages to the skin, whilst paper and plastic tapes are typically utilized in the process of adhering adhesive bandages.

5. Splints: Splints are used to offer support to damaged joints and immobilize fractured bones. Splints are also used to immobilize

shattered bones. While a patient waits for medical treatment, they may be used to help stabilize a fractured bone or wounded joint by being constructed of metal or plastic and providing support in the appropriate position.

6. Cold Packs: In order to alleviate discomfort and decrease swelling, cold packs may be applied to the affected area. Typically, they are packed with a gel or foam substance that, once frozen, may be applied to the painful region for up to 15 minutes at a time.

7. Hot Packs: The use of hot packs might assist in the alleviation of muscular pain and stiffness. Typically, they are packed with a gel or foam substance that, after warmed, may be applied to the afflicted region for up to 15 minutes at a time.

8. Gloves: When treating wounds, it is important to use gloves in order to lower the

risk of infection. When working with patients, it is standard practice to use disposable gloves, and this is an absolute must if one is attending to open wounds.

When it comes to giving basic first aid, having the appropriate materials on hand is really necessary. For the purpose of diagnosing and treating common health problems and treating minor injuries, each of the elements mentioned above is essential. In order to be ready for any kind of emergency involving first aid, it is essential to get acquainted with all of these materials and know how to use them properly.

# When to seek medical attention

Everyone should make it a priority to be knowledgeable about their own health and to be familiar with the warning signs and symptoms that may indicate the need for medical intervention.

In addition to this, it is essential to be aware of the resources that are at your disposal and to be aware of when it is necessary to seek medical treatment. If you are aware of when you should seek medical assistance, it will be easier for you to get the care you need before a health problem gets more severe.

## When It Is Necessary to Seek Medical Help

It is imperative that you get medical assistance if you encounter any of the following symptoms, since they might indicate a serious health problem:

• Significant pain that lasts for more than a few days
• A fever that lasts for more than three days
• Unexpected weight loss
• Odd bruising or bleeding
• A persistent cough
• Sudden confusion
• Chest pain
• Breathing difficulties
• Acute headache
• Weakness or numbness in the face, arm, or leg
• Severe abdominal pain
• Severe vomiting
• Severe dizziness
• Vision changes
• Difficulty swallowing
• Severe allergic reaction

In addition to the symptoms described above, it is essential to see a doctor if you have been hurt, if you have been bitten by an animal, or if you have been exposed to a disease that is infectious.

## Emergency Medical Services

It is essential to get in touch with 911 as soon as possible in the case of a medical emergency. The Emergency Medical Services (EMS) are accessible around the clock, every day of the year, to give medical attention at the times when it is most urgently required. Emergency medical services (EMS) may give help that might save a patient's life and can transfer patients to hospitals if necessary. It is essential to supply the emergency medical services dispatcher with as much information as is reasonably feasible, including the precise location of the patient, the symptoms they are experiencing, and any medical history they may have.

## When to Seek Non-Emergency Medical Care

It is imperative that you get medical attention even if you do not perceive the situation to be life-threatening even if you are suffering any of the symptoms described in the previous paragraphs. You may get the necessary medical attention from either your primary care physician or a nearby urgent care clinic. It is crucial to give the office a call ahead of time to make sure that you can schedule an appointment and that you can get the treatment that you need.

## What to Do Before requesting medical attention

It is essential to take the necessary precautions before seeking medical assistance. Be careful to keep a record of all of the medicines you are presently taking as well as any allergies you may have. It is essential that you go into the appointment with a list of questions prepared for the physician to answer. It is essential that you be aware of whatever insurance coverage you may have and that you fully comprehend the types of services that are covered by that policy.

# Conclusion

Congratulations on finishing this beginner's guide to providing first aid! You are now equipped with the necessary knowledge to provide assistance in a critical circumstance. You are able to identify a medical emergency and take appropriate action, as well as perform cardiopulmonary resuscitation (CPR) and treat a variety of common medical problems. You have also received vital information that can help you feel more assured in critical situations such as accidents or natural disasters.

We really hope that you have found this guide to be an informative resource, and we wish you the best of luck in any potential future medical crises.